C000049965

The Vibrant Vegetarian Diet Handbook

Simple and Tasty Vegetarian Recipes to Change Your Lifestyle and Boost Your Health

America Best Recipes

© Copyright 2020 - All rights reserved.

The content contained within this book may not be reproduced, duplicated or transmitted without direct written permission from the author or the publisher.

Under no circumstances will any blame or legal responsibility be held against the publisher, or author, for any damages, reparation, or monetary loss due to the information contained within this book. Either directly or indirectly.

Legal Notice:

This book is copyright protected. This book is only for personal use. You cannot amend, distribute, sell, use, quote or paraphrase any part, or the content within this book, without the consent of the author or publisher.

Disclaimer Notice:

Please note the information contained within this document is for educational and entertainment purposes only. All effort has been executed to present accurate, up to date, and reliable, complete information. No warranties of any kind are declared or implied. Readers acknowledge that the author is not engaging in the rendering of legal, financial, medical or professional advice. The content within this book has been derived from various sources. Please consult a licensed professional before attempting any techniques outlined in this book.

By reading this document, the reader agrees that under no circumstances is the author responsible for any losses, direct or indirect, which are incurred as a result of the use of information contained within this document, including, but not limited to, — errors, omissions, or inaccuracies.

Table of Contents

Breakfast.. 6

   Quinoa Pongal 6

   Barley Porridge 8

   Omelette Bites..11

   Blueberry Quinoa Muffins 14

   Mini Frittatas 17

   Potato and Zucchini Omelet.....................18

   Tomato Omelet..21

   Vegan Tropical Pina Colada Smoothie 24

   Peach Protein Bars 26

   Breakfast Tacos 28

Lunch...30

   Roasted Soy Beans and Winter Squash 30

   Chinese Roasted Button Mushrooms and Butternut Squash 33

   Roasted Button Mushrooms and Squash.................35

   Roasted Turnips and Butternut Squash 37

   Roasted Tomatoes Rutabaga and Kohlrabi Main 39

   Lemon Tofu with Garlicky Rice 41

   Baked Rainbow Carrots and Brussel Sprouts..........43

   Roasted Sweet Potato and Red Beets....................44

   Roasted Purple Cabbage and Beets.......................45

   Sichuan Style Baked Chioggia Beets and Broccoli Florets 46

Soups and Salads 48

Navy Bean and Jalapeno Pepper Soup....................48

Pigeon Peas Soup...50

Chia Seeds Tomato Soup 52

Zucchini Soup..54

Anise Seed and Cabbage Soup............................57

Green Egg Salad 59

Sesame Noodle Salad 61

Egg Salad with Beets 63

Prawn & mango salad 65

Stripy hummus salad jars.....................................67

Dinner...69

Steamed Vegetables..69

Red Thai Curry Broccoli.......................................71

Lime Ginger Green Beans.....................................73

Kale Tofu Curry...75

Potato and Broccoli Curry 77

Simple Bok Choy Stir Fry 79

Easy Broccoli Stir Fry..81

Vegetarian Alfredo Sauce 83

Vegan Fajitas..84

Grilled Summer Squash and Zucchini...................86

Sweets 88

Almond Flour Chocolate Chip Cookies 88

Keto Coconut cookies 91

Cookie dough bars no bake, keto, vegan..............93

Paleo Pumpkin Brownies 95

No bake peanut butter bars healthy.......................98

Fruity Neapolitan lolly loaf 100

Keto Breakfast Brownie Muffins........................... 102

Walnut Cardamom Bar Cookies........................... 103

Lemon-Lime Magic Cake 105

Vanilla Pudding 107

Little Jam Tarts... 108

Macadamia & Cranberry American Cookies 109

Breakfast

Quinoa Pongal

Prep time: 05 min Cooking Time: 15min Serve: 2

Ingredients

½ cup quinoa

¼ cup Moong dal

1 tablespoon coconut oil

½ teaspoon cumin

1/8 teaspoon peppercorns

1 green chili slatted

4 cashews

Few curry leaves

1 teaspoon ginger powder

A pinch Asafoetida

5 cups water

Salt and pepper to taste

Parsley leaves

Instructions:

Rinse and Soak quinoa and Moong dal for about 1 hour.

Turn on Instant Pot to Sauté mode. Once hot, add coconut oil, cumin, peppercorns, green chili, ginger powder, cashews, Asafoetida & curry leaves.

Sauté for a minute or two, until cashew turns golden brown.

Drain water from soaked dal. Next, add in soaked dal and sauté until it turns aromatic.

Add 3 cups of water, pepper powder, salt & dal. Mix well.

Close Lid of Instant Pot and turn the valve to Sealing.

Press Cancel button, turn on Manual mode (High Pressure), Set timer to 8 minutes.

Wait for natural pressure release (NPR) and open lid.

Turn on Sauté mode. Mix Pongal well, add 2 cups water and sauté until boils and slightly thickens, about 2-3 min.

Add chopped parsley leaves, mix well and serve hot.

Nutrition Facts

Calories289, Total Fat 12.9g, Saturated Fat 6.9g, Cholesterol 0mg , Sodium 163mg

Barley Porridge

Prep time: 15 min Cooking Time: 15 min Serve: 2

Ingredients

1/2 cup barley

1 tablespoon honey

1/2 teaspoon nutmeg

1/2 tablespoon unsalted butter

2 tablespoons raisins

½ cup coconut milk

2 cups water

Coconut cream for serving (optional)

Frozen berries for serving

1 cup of cold water

Directions

Add 1 cup of cold water to your Instant Pot and place a trivet inside.

Add all the ingredients to a glass dish that fits into your Instant Pot, cover with foil and place on the trivet inside Instant Pot.

Lock lid of your Instant Pot and turn the valve to Sealing.

Press Manual or Pressure Cooker button (depending on your model) and use the arrows to select 15 minutes. It will take about 5-6 minutes to come to pressure.

Once the Instant Pot beeps that the 15 minutes of cooking are done, do natural pressure release for 10 minutes. It means that you do not touch your Instant Pot for 10 minutes and do nothing.

After 10 minutes of natural pressure release are done, do a Quick-release. This will take only a few seconds.

Open the foil and mix well. If you notice that the milk is not fully absorbed, then cover with foil and let sit for another 3-5 minutes.

Transfer the cooked barley Porridge to individual serving bowls, add a few splashes of milk or cream and garnish with fruit or frozen berries if desired. Enjoy hot!

Nutrition Facts

Calories388, Total Fat 18.5g, Saturated Fat 14.9g, Cholesterol 8mg Sodium 36mg, Total Carbohydrate 53.2g, Dietary Fiber 9.8g , Total Sugars 16.5g , Protein 7.5g

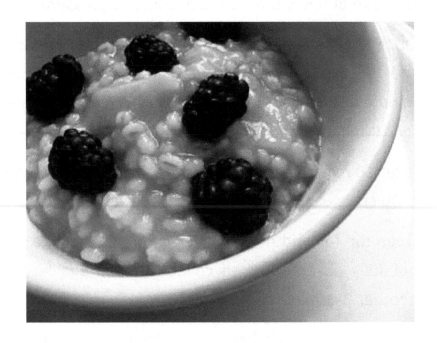

Omelette Bites

Prep time: 05 min Cooking Time: 10 min Serve: 2

Ingredients

1 whole egg, beaten

1/8 cup crumbled tofu

1/2 cup feta cheese

1 tablespoon green onions, diced and sliced

1 tablespoon green peppers, diced and sliced

1 tablespoon mushrooms, diced and sliced, small

Salt and pepper to taste

1/8 teaspoon garlic powder

1/8 teaspoon ground mustard

2 cups of water

Instructions

Whisk the egg, add tofu and feta cheese then stir until well combined.

Add vegetables, and seasonings to egg mixture. Combine them well.

Pour egg mixture into greased silicone mold. Add 2 cups of water to the Instant Pot. Set in Instant Pot on rack. Close and lock lid.

Set Instant Pot to steam on High Pressure for 8 minutes. Once done, do a 10-minute Natural-release according to your manufacturer's directions.

Set on a wire rack to cool, and then remove to a storage container.

Nutrition Facts

Calories 145, Total Fat 10.9g, Saturated Fat 6.4g, Cholesterol 115mg, Sodium 530mg, Total Carbohydrate 2.7g, Dietary Fiber 0.4g, , Total Sugars 2.1g, Protein 9.6g

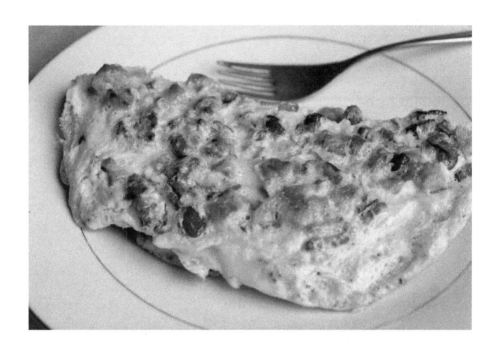

Blueberry Quinoa Muffins

Prep time: 10 min Cooking Time: 10 min Serve: 2

Ingredients

1 egg

¼ cup thick Greek yogurt

¼ cup honey

¼ tablespoon butter, melted

¼ teaspoon vanilla extract

¼ cup quinoa

1/8 cup coconut flour

¼ tablespoon baking powder

¼ teaspoon nutmeg

1/8 teaspoon salt

3/4 cup blueberries

1 cup of water

Instructions

In a large bowl combine egg, yogurt, honey, butter, and vanilla extract until smooth.

Add quinoa, coconut flour, baking powder, nutmeg, and salt and stir just until combined. Gently fold in blueberries.

Generously spray the 2 silicone molds with nonstick spray. Pour batter on molds.

Stack one of the filled molds on top of a trivet. Place 4 narrow Mason jar lids on top followed by the second silicone mould.

Pour 1 cup of water into the Instant Pot and place the trivet and filled silicone molds inside.

Lock lid and turn pressure release knob to a sealed position. Cook at High Pressure for 10 minutes.

When cooking is complete, use a Natural-release for 10 minutes and then release any remaining pressure.

Let the quinoa bites excellent if needed for handling.

Using a butter knife or spoon, scrape around each quinoa bite to release it, then turn them over on to a cooling rack or plate.

Enjoy!

Store extras in the refrigerator.

Delicious chilled or warmed back up from the fridge. Freeze beautifully as well.

Nutrition Facts

Calories 311, Total Fat 5.7g, Saturated Fat 2.2g, Cholesterol 88mg, Sodium 208mg, Total Carbohydrate 59.3g, Dietary Fiber 3.3g, Total Sugars 41.5g, Protein 9.4g

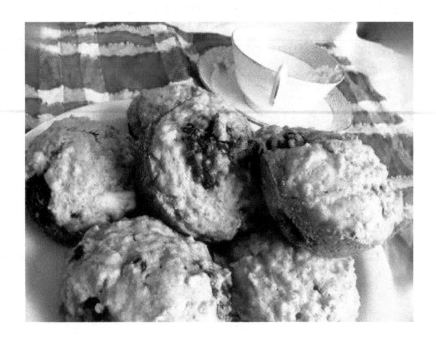

Mini Frittatas

Prep time: 10 min Cooking Time: 10 min Serve: 2

Ingredients

2 eggs

¼ teaspoon salt

1/8 teaspoon pepper

½ small red potato, small diced

¼ bell pepper, small diced

¼ small onion, small diced

1/8 cup almond milk

1/8 cup feta cheese

1 cup of water

Instructions

Add diced vegetables to on top.

Mix eggs, milk, salt and pepper. Pour the eggs over the veggies. Then sprinkle shredded feta cheese on top.

Cover each ramekin with foil, place them on the trivet with 1 cup of water on the bottom. Cook 10 minutes on

High Pressure. Once done, release the pressure using the Quick-release method. 4. Remove carefully, serve and enjoy.

Nutrition Facts

Calories161, Total Fat 10.1g, Saturated Fat 5.9g, Cholesterol 172mg , Sodium 463mg, Total Carbohydrate 10.3g, Dietary Fiber 1.5g , Total Sugars 2.8g, Protein 8.3g

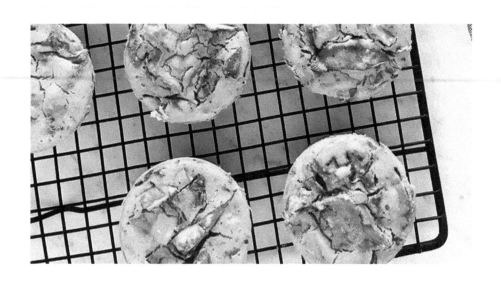

Potato and Zucchini Omelet

Preparation time: 5 minutes Cooking time: 20 minutes
Ingredients:

½ lb. potato (about 1¼ cups diced) ½ lb. zucchini (about 1½ cups diced) ⅔ cup chopped onion (1 small) 1 Tbs. butter 2 Tbs. olive oil ¼ tsp. dried dill weed ¼ tsp. dried basil, crushed ½ tsp. crushed dried red pepper salt to taste fresh-ground black pepper to taste 5 to 6 eggs butter for frying garnish sour cream

Directions:

Peel or scrub the potato and cut it in ½-inch dice. Wash, trim, and finely dice the zucchini. Drop the diced potato into boiling salted water and cook for 5 minutes, then drain it and set it aside. Cook the diced zucchini in boiling water for 3 to 4 minutes, drain, and set aside. Heat the butter and the olive oil in a medium-sized skillet and sauté the onions in it until they start to color. Add the partially cooked potato and zucchini, the dill weed, basil, crushed red pepper, and salt. Cook, stirring often, until the potatoes are just tender. Grind in some black pepper and add more salt if needed. Make either 2 medium-sized or 3 small omelets according to the directions. When the eggs are almost set, spoon some of the hot vegetables onto one side and fold the other side of the omelet over the filling. Slide the omelets out onto warm plates and serve immediately with sour cream.

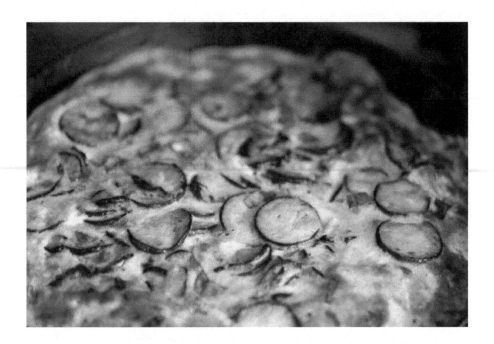

Tomato Omelet

Preparation time: 5 minutes Cooking time: 40 minutes
Servings: 3

Ingredients:

8 medium sized tomatoes 2 cloves garlic 2 bay leaves ½
tsp. dried tarragon, crushed 1 tsp. salt, and more to taste
2 Tbs. chopped fresh parsley 1 medium- sized yellow
onion 3 Tbs. olive oil ½ tsp. dried basil, crushed 5 cured
black olives, pitted and sliced coarse ground black pepper
to taste 8 to 10 eggs milk

Directions:

Peel the blanched tomatoes.

Chop the tomatoes very coarsely and put them aside in
a bowl with the salt. Chop the onion, mince the garlic,
and sauté them in the olive oil in a large skillet until they
begin to show color.

Add the bay leaves and sauté a few minutes more. Add
the tomatoes, the basil, tarragon, parsley, and sliced
olives, and cook over medium heat, stirring occasionally,
until the sauce is thick. It should take about 40 to 45
minutes. Make individual omelets according to the

directions. Spoon on some of the hot Provençale sauce just when the eggs are nearly set.

Peel the blanched tomatoes. Chop the tomatoes very coarsely and put them aside in a bowl with the salt. Chop the onion, mince the garlic, and sauté them in the olive oil in a large skillet until they begin to show color.

Add the bay leaves and sauté a few minutes more. Add the tomatoes, the basil, tarragon, parsley, and sliced olives, and cook over medium heat, stirring occasionally, until the sauce is thick. It should take about 40 to 45 minutes.

Make individual omelets according to the directions. Spoon on some of the hot Provençale sauce just when the eggs are nearly set, and fold the omelets over the sauce. Serve.

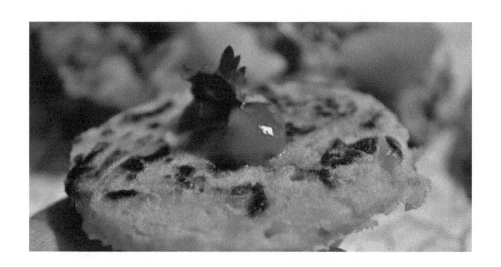

Vegan Tropical Pina Colada Smoothie

Preparation time: 5 minutes Cooking time: 0 minutes 1 smoothie.

Ingredients:

¾ cup soymilk

½ cup coconut milk

1 banana 1 ½ tbsp. ground flax seed

1 tsp. vanilla

1 cup pineapple

1 tbsp. agave nectar

3 ice cubes

Directions:

Blend all the ingredients to achieve your desired smoothie consistency.

Enjoy!

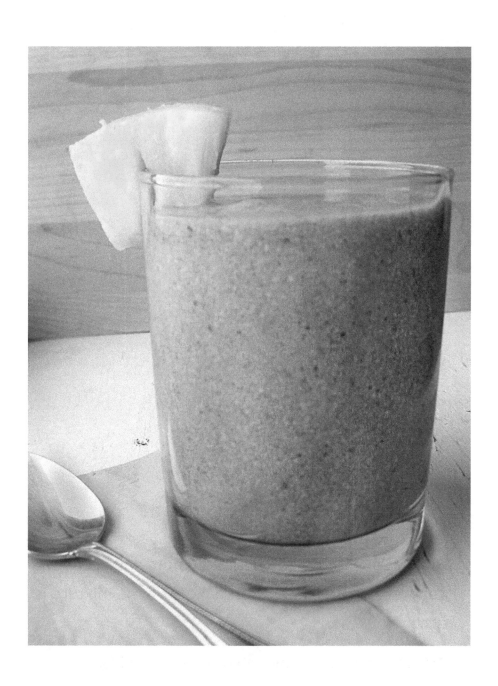

Peach Protein Bars

Servings: 6 Preparation Time: 60 min

Ingredients:

1 cup flax seeds

½ cup peanuts

¼ cup hemp seeds

15g dehydrated peaches

2 tbsp. psyllium husk

¼ tsp. stevia

½ tsp. salt

1¼ cup water

Directions:

Preheat oven at 350°F. Grind up nuts and seeds with ½ cup water in a blender, but make sure the mixture is not acceptable.

Transfer and combine mixture with psyllium husk and cinnamon in a mixing bowl. Crush the dehydrated peaches into small bits and add to mixing bowl.

Stir in the remaining water and salt until all ingredients are combined.

Spread the mixture out on a baking sheet lined with parchment paper, and make sure the dough is about ¼ inch thick.

Bake for 45 minutes, remove around 30 minutes to cut the dough carefully in six pieces, and bake for another 15 minutes. Remove from oven and cool for 30 minutes. Can be stored for a week or frozen up to two months.

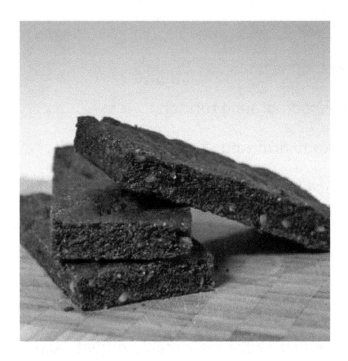

Breakfast Tacos

Preparation Time: 10 minutes Cooking time: 6 minutes
Servings: 4

Ingredients

½ cup grape tomatoes, quartered

1 avocado, sliced

8 corn tortillas

Freshly ground black pepper

¼ teaspoon salt

¼ teaspoon cumin

¼ teaspoon ground turmeric

1 package firm tofu

1 garlic clove, minced

1 red pepper, diced 1 teaspoon olive oil

Directions:

Heat oil in a skillet over medium heat. Add in garlic and
red pepper and sauté for around 2 minutes. Using your

hands, crumble the tofu and add into the pan; and then add the seasonings.

Cook for around 5 minutes making sure that you stir frequently. Taste and adjust the seasonings then apportion it and store in containers for the week.

When you want to serve, simply put the scramble on tortillas, add any other toppings and enjoy.

Lunch
Roasted Soy Beans and Winter Squash

Ingredients

2 (15 ounces) cans soy beans, rinsed and drained

1/2 winter squash - peeled, seeded, and cut into 1-inch pieces

1 red onion, diced

1 sweet potato, peeled and cut into 1-inch cubes

2 large carrots, cut into 1 inch pieces

3 medium potatoes, cut into 1-inch pieces

4 tablespoons extra virgin oil

Seasoning ingredients

1 teaspoon salt

1/2 teaspoon ground black pepper

1 teaspoon onion powder

1 teaspoon dried basil

1 teaspoon Italian seasoning

Garnishing Ingredients

2 green onions, chopped (optional)

Directions:

Preheat your oven to 350 degrees F. Grease your
baking pan. Combine the beans, squash, onion, sweet
potato, carrots, and russet potatoes on the prepared
sheet pan. Drizzle with the oil and toss to coat.
Combine the seasoning ingredients in a bowl. Sprinkle
them over the vegetables on the pan and toss to coat
with seasonings. Bake in the oven for 25 minutes. Stir
frequently until vegetables are soft and lightly browned
and beans are crisp, for about 20 to 25 minutes more.
Season with more salt and black pepper to taste, top
with the green onion before serving.

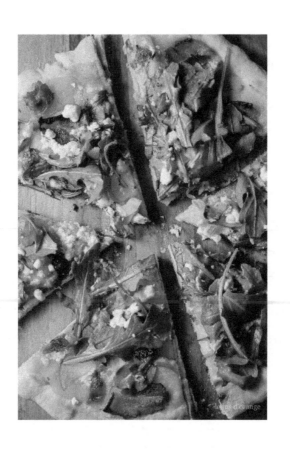

Chinese Roasted Button Mushrooms and Butternut Squash

Ingredients

2 (15 ounces) cans button mushrooms, sliced and drained

1/2 butternut squash -peeled, seeded, and cut into 1-inch pieces

1 red onion, diced

2 large carrots, cut into 1 inch pieces

3 medium turnips, cut into 1-inch pieces

3 tablespoons sesame oil

Seasoning ingredients

1 teaspoon salt

1/2 teaspoon ground black pepper

1 teaspoon onion powder

2 teaspoon garlic powder

1 teaspoon Sichuan peppercorns

1 teaspoon Chinese five-spice powder

Garnishing Ingredients

2 green onions, chopped (optional)

Directions:

Preheat your oven to 350 degrees F. Grease your baking pan. Combine the main ingredients on the prepared sheet pan. Drizzle with the oil and toss to coat. Combine the seasoning ingredients in a bowl. Sprinkle them over the vegetables on the pan and toss to coat with seasonings. Bake in the oven for 25 minutes. Stir frequently until vegetables are soft and lightly browned and chickpeas are crisp, for about 20 to 25 minutes more. Season with more salt and black pepper to taste, top with the green onion before serving.

Roasted Button Mushrooms and Squash

Ingredients

2 (15 ounce) cans button mushrooms, rinsed and drained

1/2 summer squash peeled, seeded, and cut into 1-inch pieces

1 red onion, diced

2 large turnips, cut into 1 inch pieces

2 large parsnips, cut into 1 inch pieces

3 medium potatoes, cut into 1-inch pieces

3 tablespoons butter

Seasoning ingredients

1 teaspoon salt

1/2 teaspoon ground black pepper

1 teaspoon onion powder

2 teaspoon garlic powder

1 teaspoon Herbs de Provence

Garnishing Ingredients

2 sprigs of thyme, chopped (optional)

Directions:

Preheat your oven to 350 degrees F. Grease your baking pan. Combine the main ingredients on the prepared sheet pan. Drizzle with the melted butter or margarine and toss to coat. Combine the seasoning ingredients in a bowl. Sprinkle them over the vegetables on the pan and toss to coat with seasonings. Bake in the oven for 25 minutes. Stir frequently until vegetables are soft and lightly browned and chickpeas are crisp, for about 20 to 25 minutes more. Season with more salt and black pepper to taste, top with thyme before serving.

Roasted Turnips and Butternut Squash

Ingredients

3   medium tomatoes, cut into 1-inch pieces

1/2 butternut squash - peeled, seeded, and cut into 1-inch pieces

1 red onion, diced

1 turnip, peeled, and cut into 1-inch cubes

2 large carrots, cut into 1 inch pieces

2 large kohlrabi, cut into 1 inch pieces

3 tablespoons extra virgin olive oil

Seasoning ingredients

1 teaspoon salt

1/2 teaspoon ground black pepper

1 teaspoon onion powder

2 teaspoon garlic powder

1 teaspoon dried thyme

Garnishing Ingredients

2 sprigs fresh thyme, chopped (optional)

Directions:

Preheat your oven to 350 degrees F. Grease your baking pan. Combine the main ingredients on the prepared sheet pan. Drizzle with the oil and toss to coat. Combine the seasoning ingredients in a bowl. Sprinkle them over the vegetables on the pan and toss to coat with seasonings. Bake in the oven for 25 minutes. Stir frequently until vegetables are soft and lightly browned and chickpeas are crisp, for about 20 to 25 minutes more. Season with more salt and black pepper to taste, top with the thyme before serving.

Roasted Tomatoes Rutabaga and Kohlrabi Main

Ingredients

3 large tomatoes, cut into 1-inch pieces

3 red onion, diced

1 rutabaga, peeled and cut into 1-inch cubes

2 large carrots, cut into 1 inch pieces

3 medium kohlrabi, cut into 1-inch pieces

3 tablespoons extra virgin olive oil

Seasoning ingredients

1 teaspoon salt

1/2 teaspoon ground black pepper

1 teaspoon onion powder

2 teaspoon garlic powder

1 teaspoon Spanish paprika

1 teaspoon cumin

Garnishing Ingredients

2 sprigs parsley, chopped (optional)

Directions:

Preheat your oven to 350 degrees F. Grease your baking pan. Combine the main ingredients on the prepared sheet pan. Drizzle with the oil and toss to coat. Combine the seasoning ingredients in a bowl. Sprinkle them over the vegetables on the pan and toss to coat with seasonings. Bake in the oven for

25 minutes. Stir frequently until vegetables are soft, for about 20 to 25 minutes more. Season with more salt and black pepper to taste, top with the parsley before serving.

Lemon Tofu with Garlicky Rice

Prep time: 15 min Cooking Time: 20 min serve: 2

Ingredients

½ cup jasmine rice

½ teaspoon garlic, grated

1 cup vegetable stock

1 lemon, cut into wheels

1 cup tofu

Salt to taste

Freshly ground black pepper

1 tablespoon coconut oil

1/8 cup freshly chopped mint

Instructions

Start the Instant Pot on Sauté mode and heat it. Add coconut oil; add garlic powder. Add lemon and tofu mix well.

41

Add the jasmine rice and vegetable stock to the Instant Pot. Stir the salt, pepper in the Instant Pot.

Change the Instant Pot setting to Manual and cook for 4 minutes at High Pressure.

When the Instant Pot beeps, do a 10-minute natural pressure release. This means let the pressure release naturally for 10 minutes, then release the remaining pressure manually.

Serve with chopped mint.

Nutrition Facts

Calories 334, Total Fat 12.2g, Saturated Fat 7g, Cholesterol 0mg, Sodium 120mg, Total Carbohydrate 42g, Dietary Fiber 4.6g, Total Sugars 1.9g, Protein 14.1g

Baked Rainbow Carrots and Brussel Sprouts

Ingredients

1 ½ cups Brussels sprouts, trimmed

1 cup large potato chunks

1 cup large rainbow carrot chunks

1 ½ cup broccoli florets

1 cup cubed red beets

1/2 cup red onion chunks

2 tablespoons extra-virgin olive oil

Salt and ground black pepper to taste

Directions:

Preheat your oven to 425 degrees F (220 degrees C). Set the rack to the second-lowest level in the oven. Pour some lightly salted water into a bowl. Submerge the Brussels sprouts in salted water for 15 minutes and drain. Place the rest of the ingredients together in a bowl. Spread the vegetables in a single layer onto a baking pan. Roast in the oven until the vegetables start to brown and cook through for about 45 minutes.

Roasted Sweet Potato and Red Beets

Ingredients

1 ½ cups Brussels sprouts, trimmed

1 cup large sweet potato chunks

1 cup large carrot chunks

1 ½ cup broccoli florets

1 cup cubed red beets

1/2 cup yellow onion chunks

2 tablespoons sesame seed oil

Salt and ground black pepper to taste

Directions:

Preheat your oven to 425 degrees F (220 degrees C). Set the rack to the second-lowest level in the oven. Pour some lightly salted water into a bowl. Submerge the Brussels sprouts in salted water for 15 minutes and drain. Place the rest of the ingredients together in a bowl. Spread the vegetables in a single layer onto a baking pan. Roast in the oven until the vegetables start to brown and cook through for about 45 minutes.

Roasted Purple Cabbage and Beets

Ingredients

1 ½ cups purple cabbage, trimmed

1 cup large potato chunks

1 cup large carrot chunks

1 ½ cup cauliflower florets

1 cup cubed red beets

1/2 cup Vidalia onion chunks

2 tablespoons extra-virgin olive oil

Sea salt and ground black pepper to taste

Directions:

Preheat your oven to 425 degrees F (220 degrees C). Set the rack to the second-lowest level in the oven. Pour some lightly salted water into a bowl. Submerge the purple cabbage in salted water for 15 minutes and drain. Place the rest of the ingredients together in a bowl. Spread the vegetables in a single layer onto a baking pan. Roast in the oven until the vegetables start to brown and cook through for about 45 minutes.

Sichuan Style Baked Chioggia Beets and Broccoli Florets

Ingredients

1 ½ cups Brussels sprouts, trimmed

1 cup broccoli florets

1 cup Chioggia beets, cut into chunks

1 ½ cup cauliflower florets

1 cup button mushrooms, sliced

1/2 cup red onion chunks

2 tablespoons sesame oil

½ tsp. Sichuan peppercorns

Salt ground black pepper to taste

Directions:

Preheat your oven to 425 degrees F (220 degrees C). Set the rack to the second-lowest level in the oven. Pour some lightly salted water into a bowl. Submerge the Brussels sprouts in salted water for 15 minutes and drain. Place the rest of the ingredients together in a bowl. Spread the vegetables in a single layer onto a baking pan. Roast in the oven until the vegetables start to brown and cook through for about 45 minutes.

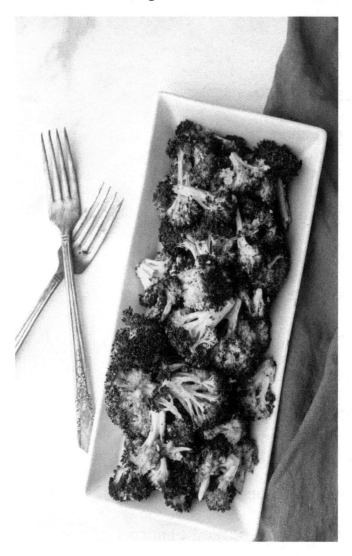

Soups and Salads

Navy Bean and Jalapeno Pepper Soup

Ingredients:

1 teaspoon olive oil

1/2 cup chopped red onions

4 cloves garlic, minced

1 cup vegetable broth

1 cup vegetable stock

1 cup salsa

1 14-ounce can navy beans

1 green bell pepper, chopped

1 jalapeno pepper, coarsely chopped

1/2 teaspoon sea salt

1 avocado, chopped

1/2 cup loosely-packed cilantro

Directions:

Optional: 1/2 cup crumbled corn tortilla chips Add olive oil to a pan and heat it to medium. Add red onions and garlic to the saucepan and sauté until softened. Add the stock, salsa, bell peppers, jalapeno, beans, and sea salt. Bring to a boil over high heat. Reduce to low and simmer for 5 minutes. Garnish with half of the avocado, cilantro, and tortilla chips.

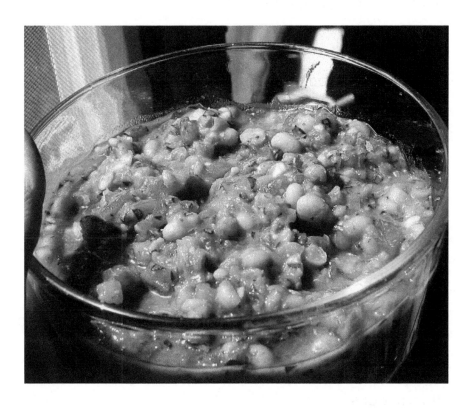

Pigeon Peas Soup

(Prep time: 10 min| Cooking Time: 20 min| Serve: 2)

Ingredients

½ tablespoon butter

1 tablespoon fresh ginger, peeled and finely chopped

1 tablespoon garlic, minced

½ large onion, finely chopped

1 parsnip, peeled and finely diced

½ cup broccoli

½ teaspoon salt

½ cup unsweetened soy milk

2 cups water

½ cup dried pigeon peas, picked over and rinsed

1 tablespoon finely chopped parsley leaves for garnish

Instructions

In an Instant Pot, press Sauté and melt the butter. Add the onion, ginger, garlic, parsnip, and broccoli. Sauté until the vegetables are tender, about 5 minutes.

Add the water, soy milk, pigeon peas and season with salt and lock lid in place, and turn the valve to Sealing. Press Manual or Pressure Cooker; cook at High Pressure 15 minutes. When cooking is complete, use Natural-release for 10 minutes, then release remaining pressure. Let the soup cool slightly, then puree the soup in a blender until smooth.

Ladle soup into 2 bowls and garnish with chopped parsley.

Nutrition Facts

Calories 159, Total Fat 4.3g, Saturated Fat 2g, Cholesterol 8mg, Sodium 649mg, Total Carbohydrate

25.3g, Dietary Fiber 5.9g, Total Sugars 5.7g, Protein 6.1g

Chia Seeds Tomato Soup

(Prep time: 05 min| Cooking Time: 10 min| Serve: 2)

Ingredients

4 tomatoes, chopped

½ cup chia seeds

½ tablespoon butter

½ teaspoon garlic powder

½ small onion, roughly chopped

½ small zucchini, roughly chopped

1 1/2 cups vegetable broth

Salt and black pepper to taste

Instructions

Put Instant Pot on Sauté mode High and when hot, add the butter. Now add garlic powder and onion to fry, sauté well till onions soften.

Now add zucchini and chia seeds and fry for a minute.

Add in the tomatoes and mix well. Fry for 3 mines.

Now add in broth, salt, and pepper. Mix them well.

Lock lid in place and turn the valve to Sealing. Do Manual Low Pressure for 2 min. 7. When cooking is complete, use Natural-release for 10 minutes, then release remaining pressure. 8. Blend the chia seeds tomato mixture into a smooth puree.

If desired, adjust the consistency of the soup. Serve hot.

Nutrition Facts

Calories116, Total Fat 5.8g, Saturated Fat 2.2g, Cholesterol 8mg, Sodium 303mg, Total Carbohydrate 13.5g, Dietary Fiber 5.4g, Total Sugars 6.4g, Protein 4.7g

Zucchini Soup

(Prep time: 05 min| Cooking Time: 10 min| Serve: 2)

Ingredients

¼ medium onion diced

1 teaspoon coconut oil

1 teaspoon garlic powder

2 zucchini, peeled and cut into 4-inch chunks

½ sweet potato

½ cup almond milk

2 cups vegetable broth

1 teaspoon salt

½ teaspoon pepper

Instructions

Select the Sauté function to heat the Instant Pot. When the pot displays —Hot‖, add the coconut oil, onion, and garlic powder. Sauté until the onion softens. Press Cancel to turn off the sauté function.

Add the zucchini, sweet potato, almond milk, broth, salt, and pepper. Stir well. Lock lid in place and turn the valve to Sealing. Press the Pressure Cooker button and set the time to 10 minutes.

Once cooking is complete, turn the valve to the Venting position to release the pressure. When all the pressure is released, carefully remove the lid.

Stir the soup. Blend with an immersion blender or in batches in a stand blender until smooth.

Serve hot.

Nutrition Facts

Calories277, Total Fat 16.5g, Saturated Fat 13.2g, Cholesterol 0mg, Sodium 1986mg, Total Carbohydrate 26g, Dietary Fiber 7.2g, Total Sugars 12.3g, Protein 12.1g

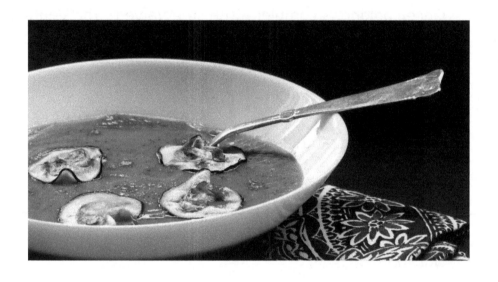

Anise Seed and Cabbage Soup

(Prep time: 10 min| Cooking Time: 15 min| Serve: 2)

Ingredients

½ tablespoon olive oil

½ onion

½ teaspoon garlic minced

½ tablespoon anise seed

½ pound cabbage

½ cup almond milk

2 cups vegetable broth

½ teaspoon salt and black pepper for serving

Instructions

Select the Sauté function to heat the Instant Pot. When the pot displays —Hot‖, add the olive oil, onion, and garlic. Sauté until the onion softens.

Add the cabbage, anise seed, almond milk, broth, salt, and pepper. Stir well. Lock lid in place and turn the valve to Sealing. Press the Pressure Cooker button and set the time to10 minutes.

Once cooking is complete, turn the valve to the Venting position to release the pressure. When all the pressure is released, carefully remove the lid.

Use a standing blender or an immersion blender to puree the soup to a smooth, creamy consistency.

Serve.

Nutrition Facts

Calories253, Total Fat 19.6g, Saturated Fat 13.6g, Cholesterol 0mg, Sodium 1376mg, Total Carbohydrate 14.5g, Dietary Fiber 5g, Total Sugars 7.5g, Protein 8.3g

Green Egg Salad

(Prep time: 15 min| Cooking Time: 15 min | serve: 2)

Ingredients

2 eggs

½ avocados, peeled, pitted, and mashed

¼ cups chopped kale

1 leek, chopped

¼ cup plain yogurt

1 pinch red pepper flakes, or to taste

½ teaspoon garlic powder

Black pepper to taste

1 cup water

Instructions

Pour the water into the Instant Pot. Place a steamer basket or the trivet in the pot. Carefully arrange eggs in the steamer basket. Secure the lid on the pot. Close the pressure-release valve. For hard-cooked eggs, select Manual and Cook at Low Pressure for 5 minutes. When cooking time is complete, use a Natural Release to depressurize. Remove the lid from the pot and gently place eggs in a bowl of cool water.

Mash eggs and avocado together in a bowl. Stir kale, leeks, and yogurt into the egg mixture; season with red pepper flakes, garlic powder, and black pepper.

Nutrition Facts

Calories 221, Total Fat 14.7g, Saturated Fat 3.8g, Cholesterol 166mg, Sodium 99mg, Total Carbohydrate 14.5g, Dietary Fiber 4.4g, Total Sugars 4.7g, Protein 9.3g

Sesame Noodle Salad

(Prep time: 15 min| Cooking Time: 10 min | serve: 2)

Ingredients

¼ cup angel hair pasta

½ tablespoon sesame oil

½ tablespoon soy sauce

½ tablespoon hot chili sauce

¼ teaspoon honey

1 teaspoon sesame seeds

1 celery, chopped

1 yellow bell pepper, diced

1 cup water

Instructions

In Instant Pot. Add angel hair, pasta, and water. Cover the Instant Pot and lock it.

Set the Manual or Pressure Cook timer for 10 minutes.

Whisk together the sesame oil, soy sauce, chili sauce, and honey in a large bowl. Toss the pasta in the dressing, then sprinkle with sesame seeds, celery, and bell pepper. Serve warm, or cover and refrigerate for a cold salad.

Nutrition Facts

Calories 110, Total Fat 4.7g, Saturated Fat 0.6g, Cholesterol 12mg, Sodium

333mg, Total Carbohydrate

15g, Dietary Fiber 1.2g, Total Sugars 4g, Protein 3g

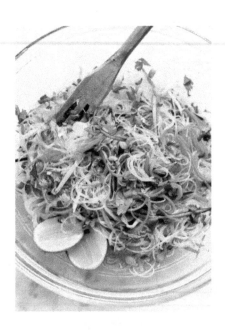

Egg Salad with Beets

(Prep time: 15 min| Cooking Time: 10 min | serve: 2)

Ingredients

2 small beets

4 eggs

½ apple, cored and diced

¼ cup chopped almond

½ tablespoon Greek yogurt

2 teaspoons chopped fresh parsley

Salt to taste

1 cup water

Instructions

Pour the water into the Instant Pot. Place a steamer basket or the trivet in the pot. Carefully arrange eggs in the steamer basket. Secure the lid on the pot. Close the pressure-release valve. For hard-cooked eggs, select

Manual and cook at Low Pressure for 5 minutes. When cooking time is complete, use a Natural Release to depressurize. Remove the lid from the Instant Pot and gently place eggs in a bowl of cool water. Place eggs, apple, yogurt, parsley, and salt into the bowl with beets; toss to combine.

Nutrition Facts

Calories 318, Total Fat 16g, Saturated Fat 4g, Cholesterol 330mg, Sodium 295mg, Total Carbohydrate 23g, Dietary Fiber 4.9g, Total Sugars 17g, Protein 20.5g

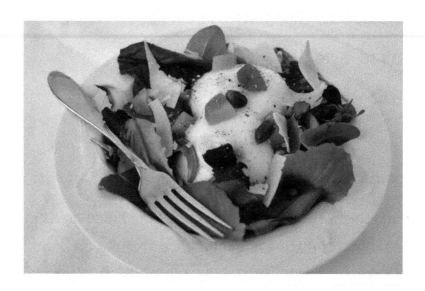

Prawn & mango salad

Prep:10 mins No-cook Easy Serves 2

Ingredients

½ avocado, peeled and cut into cubes, see tip, below left

a squeeze of lemon juice

50g small cooked prawns

1 mango cheek, peeled and cut into cubes

4 cherry tomatoes, halved

finger-sized piece cucumber, chopped

handful baby spinach leaves

a couple of mint leaves, very finely shredded

1-2 tsp sweet chili sauce

Directions:

1 Mix the avocado with the lemon juice, then toss with the prawns, mango, tomatoes, cucumber, spinach, and

mint. Pack into a lunchbox and drizzle over the sweet chili sauce, then chill until ready to eat.

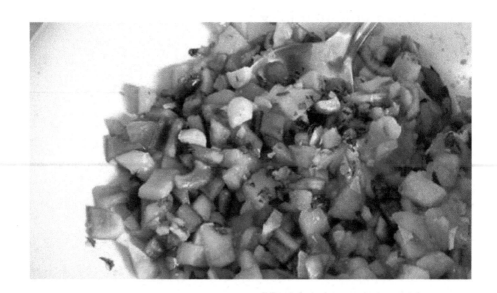

Stripy hummus salad jars

Prep: 15 mins No-cook Easy 6 jars

Ingredients

140g frozen soya beans or peas

200g tub hummus (reserve 2 tbsp for the dressing)

2 red peppers (or a mixture of colors) finely chopped

Half cucumber, finely chopped

200g cherry tomatoes, quartered

2 large carrots

small pack basil

2 large carrots, peeled and grated

4 tbsp pumpkin seeds (optional) For the dressing

zest and juice 1 lemon

1 tbsp clear honey

2 tbsp hummus (from the tub, above)

Directions:

1 First, make the dressing. Put the ingredients in a jam jar with 1 tbsp water. Screw on the lid and shake well. Set aside. 2 Bring a small pan of water to the boil, add the beans or peas and cook for 1 min until tender. Drain and run under cold water until cool. Divide the remaining hummus between 6 large jam jars. Top with the drained soya beans or peas, peppers, cucumber, tomatoes, basil leaves, carrots, and pumpkin seeds, if using. Screw on the lids and chill until needed. Will keep in the fridge for 24 hrs. 3 When ready to serve, pass around the jars and let everyone pour over a little dressing.

Dinner

Steamed Vegetables

(Prep time: 10 min |Cooking Time: 10 min | serve: 2)

Ingredients

3/4 cup water

½ head broccoli, chopped

½ head cauliflower, chopped

1 zucchini, chopped

½ red pepper, chopped

½ yellow pepper, chopped

¼ teaspoon salt

1/8 teaspoon pepper

Instructions

Add the 3/4 cup of water to the bottom of the Instant Pot and then place the trivet inside the inner pot. Add veggies, then place the lid on Instant Pot and make sure valve is set to —Sealing‖. Press the Pressure Cook button and set it to High, then cook for 0 minutes. Yes, zero minutes is all that's needed to steam! The Instant Pot will take about 5-10 minutes to come to pressure, then notify you it's done by beeping. Press the Cancel button, then do a quick release of the pressure on the Instant Pot by flicking the switch at the top with a spoon. Open the lid when the pressure gauge has dropped, and the lid opens easily. Season veggies if desired, then serve and enjoy!

Nutrition Facts

Calories 62, Total Fat 0.5g, Saturated Fat 0.1g, Cholesterol 0mg, Sodium 42mg, Total Carbohydrate

13.5g, Dietary Fiber 4.2g, Total Sugars 5.2g, Protein 3.9g

Red Thai Curry Broccoli

(Prep time: 10 min |Cooking Time: 02 min | serve: 2)

Ingredients

1 cup coconut milk

½ cup water

1 tablespoon red curry paste

1 teaspoon garlic, minced

½ teaspoon salt, plus more as needed

¼ teaspoon ginger powder

1 tablespoon onions

1/8 teaspoon chili powder

½ bell pepper any color, thinly sliced

2 cups broccoli, cut into bite-size pieces

2 cups diced tomatoes and liquid

Freshly ground black pepper

Instructions

In your Instant Pot, stir together the coconut milk, water, red curry paste, minced garlic, salt, ginger powder, onion, and chili powder. Add the bell pepper, broccoli, and tomatoes, and stir again. Lock the lid and turn the steam release handle to Sealing. Using the Manual or Pressure Cook function, set the cooker to High Pressure for 2 minutes.

When the cooking time is complete, quickly release the pressure. Carefully remove the lid and give the whole thing a good stir. Taste and season with more salt and pepper, as needed. Serve with rice.

Nutrition Facts

Calories 190, Total Fat 4.8g, Saturated Fat 1g, Cholesterol 0mg, Sodium 987mg, Total Carbohydrate 29.9g, Dietary Fiber 7.9g, Total Sugars 15.4g, Protein 9.2g

Lime Ginger Green Beans

(Prep time: 5 min |Cooking Time: 0 min | serve: 2)

Ingredients

2 cups green beans, cut into 4 inches

1 cup water

1 tablespoon vegetable oil

2 teaspoons freshly squeezed lime juice

½ teaspoon salt

1 teaspoon ginger powder

Instructions

Place the green beans in a steamer basket and put the basket into the Instant Pot. Add the water. Lock the lid and turn the steam release handle to Sealing. Using the Manual or Pressure Cook function, set the cooker to Low Pressure for 0 minutes. When the cooking time is complete, quickly release the pressure. In a serving bowl, stir together the vegetable oil, lime juice, salt, and ginger powder. Carefully remove the lid and add the green beans to the bowl. Toss to combine. Taste and add the remaining lemon juice or ginger, as needed.

Nutrition Facts

Calories 121, Total Fat 7g, Saturated Fat 1.4g, Cholesterol 0mg, Sodium 593mg, Total Carbohydrate 12.2g, Dietary Fiber 4.1g, Total Sugars 2.3g, Protein 2.3g

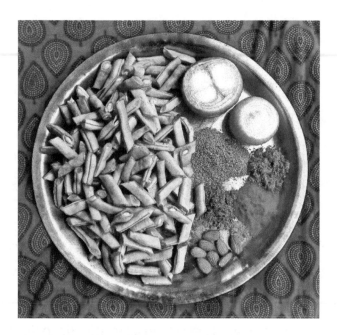

Kale Tofu Curry

(Prep time: 5 min |Cooking Time: 20 min | serve: 2)

Ingredients

1 1/2 tablespoons coconut oil

¼ onion, finely chopped

½ green chili, finely chopped

½ tablespoon ginger and garlic paste

2 cups kale

1/2 cup water

1 cup tofu cubes

2 tablespoons coconut cream to garnish

1 medium tomato, finely chopped

½ tablespoon cumin seeds

1 tablespoon coriander powder

1 teaspoon Garam masala powder

Red chili powder to taste

Instructions

Press Sauté mode on High Pressure. Add coconut oil and let it get hot; add cumin seeds and fry well. Add onions and green chili, sauté, then add tomatoes, fry till mushy. Add in the spice powders and salt, mix well, then add in the kale, water, and mix. Turn off Sauté mode. Make sure the vent is set to —Sealing‖. Using the Manual function, set the cooker to High Pressure for 2 minutes and quickly release after 2 minutes in Warm mode. Now grind the kale onion tomato mix using a hand blender or a regular blender to a fine paste. Add in more water to desired consistency and press Sauté mode on High Pressure for 5 minutes or so. Add Garam masala and mix, then add in the tofu cubes and simmer for 2-4 minutes. Serve with coconut cream if desired.

Nutrition Facts

Calories 266, Total Fat 13.7g, Saturated Fat 9g, Cholesterol 0mg, Sodium 131mg, Total Carbohydrate

30.2g, Dietary Fiber 2.2g, Total Sugars 12.1g, Protein 5.5g

Potato and Broccoli Curry

(Prep time: 10 min |Cooking Time: 10 min | serve: 2)

Ingredients

1 tablespoon avocado oil

1 teaspoon mustard seed

1 onion, chopped

½ tablespoon hot curry powder

1 cup ripe tomatoes

2 potatoes, unpeeled and cut

Salt and pepper

1 medium broccoli cut into large (3-inch) florets, stalk, and core discarded

Instructions

Put the avocado oil in the Instant Pot, select Sauté, and adjust to Normal/Medium heat. When the oil is hot, add the mustard seeds and cook until they have popped and turned gray for about 1 minute. Add the onions and curry powder and cook, frequently stirring, until the onions are tender, about 4 minutes. Add the tomatoes and cook until they break down a bit, about 2 minutes.

Add the potatoes, 1/2 cup water, 1 teaspoon salt, and several grinds of pepper and stir into the tomato mixture. Place the broccoli florets on top of the potato mixture, but don't stir. Lock the lid, select the Pressure Cook function, and adjust to Low Pressure for 2 minutes. Make sure the steam valve is in the ―Sealing‖. When the cooking time is up, quickly release the pressure. Pour the mixture into a large serving bowl and break up the broccoli a bit with a spoon. Serve immediately.

Nutrition Facts

Calories 226, Total Fat 2.4g, Saturated Fat 0.3g, Cholesterol 0mg, Sodium 122mg, Total Carbohydrate

44.3g, Dietary Fiber 7.1g, Total Sugars 6.8g, Protein 6.9g

Simple Bok Choy Stir Fry

Ingredients

1 bunch bok choy, rinsed and drained

1/2 tsp. salt

1/2 tsp. Chinese chili garlic paste

1 Tbsp. sesame oil

1/4 cup diced green pepper

1/4 cup diced red onion

3 clove garlic, minced

1 Tbsp. chopped flat-leaf parsley

1 Tbsp. vegan bacon bits (optional)

Pepper, to taste (optional)

Directions:

In a bowl, mix the bok choy, chili garlic paste & salt thoroughly. Heat the oil over medium heat and add the pepper, onion, and garlic. Stir fry for 2 1/2 minutes, or until just softened. Add the tofu mixture and cook for

15 minutes. Garnish with parsley, soy bacon pieces, and
pepper.

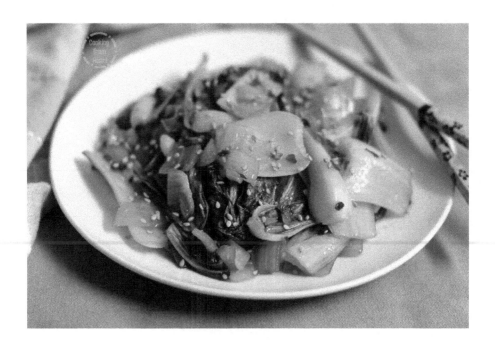

Easy Broccoli Stir Fry

Ingredients

20 pcs. broccoli, rinsed, rinsed, and drained

Juice of 1/2 lemon

1/2 tsp. salt

1 Tbsp. extra virgin olive oil

1/4 cup diced green pepper

1/4 cup diced red onion

3 clove garlic, minced

1 Tbsp. chopped flat-leaf parsley

1 Tbsp. vegan bacon bits (optional)

Pepper, to taste (optional)

In a bowl, mix the broccoli, lemon juice, and salt
thoroughly.

Directions:

Heat the oil over medium heat and add the pepper,
onion, and garlic. Stir fry for 2 1/2 minutes, or until just

softened. Add the tofu mixture and cook for 15 minutes. Garnish with parsley, soy bacon pieces, and pepper.

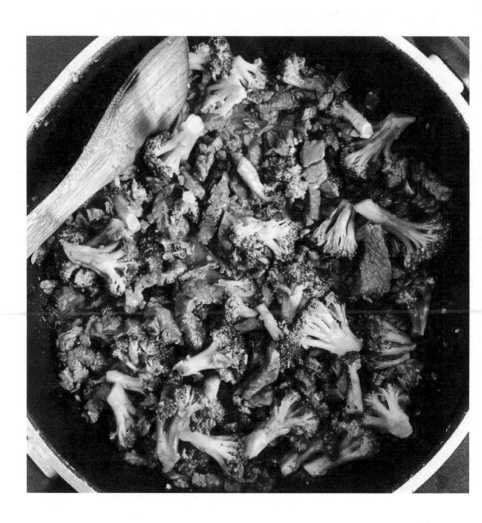

Vegetarian Alfredo Sauce

Ingredients

1/4 cup butter

3 cloves garlic, minced

2 cups cooked white beans, rinsed and drained

1 1/2 cups unsweetened almond milk

Sea salt and pepper, to taste

Parsley (optional)

Directions:

Melt the butter on low heat. Add the garlic and cook for 2 ½ minutes. Transfer to a food processor, add the beans and 1 cup of almond milk. Blend until smooth. Pour the sauce into the pan over low heat and season with salt and pepper. Add the parsley. Cook until warm.

Vegan Fajitas

Ingredients

1 can Refried Beans (15oz)

1 can Lima Beans (15oz), drained and rinsed

1/4 cup Salsa

1 Red Onion sliced into strips

1 Green Bell Pepper sliced into strips

2 Tbsp Lime Juice

2 tsp Fajita Spice Mix (see below) Tortillas Fajita Mix

1 Tbsp. Corn Starch

2 tsp Chili Powder

1 tsp Spanish Paprika

1 tsp honey

1/2 tsp Sea salt

1/2 teaspoon Onion Powder

1/2 teaspoon Garlic Powder

1/2 teaspoon Ground Cumin

1/8 teaspoon Cayenne Pepper

Directions:

Simmer salsa and refried beans until warm. Add and mix the fajita) mix ingredients in a small bowl and leave 2 tsp. Behind. Sauté the onion, pepper, and 2 tsp of Spice Mix in water and lime juice. Continue until liquid evaporates and vegetables start to brown Layer the beans in the middle of the tortilla. Layer with the stir-fried veggies and toppings. Roll it up and serve.

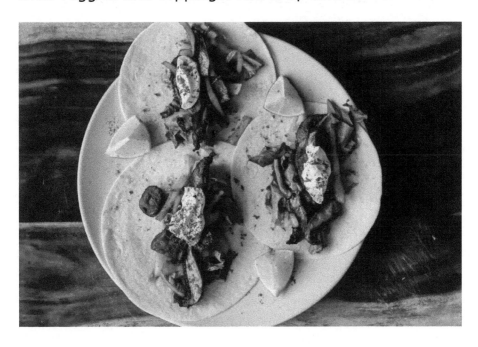

Grilled Summer Squash and Zucchini

Ingredients

1 summer squash, peeled and sliced lengthwise

1 lb zucchini, sliced lengthwise into shorter sticks

1 lb yellow bell peppers, sliced into wide strips

10 Broccolini Florets

10 pcs. Brussel Sprouts

1 large red onion, cut into 1/2 inch thick rounds

1/3 cup Italian parsley or basil, finely chopped

Dressing:

6 tbsp. extra virgin olive oil

Sea salt, to taste

3 tbsp. apple cider vinegar

1 tbsp. honey

Directions:

Egg-free mayonnaise Combine all of the dressing ingredients thoroughly. Preheat your grill to low heat

86

and grease the grates. Layer the vegetable grill for 12 minutes per side until tender, flipping once. Brush with the marinade/ dressing ingredients

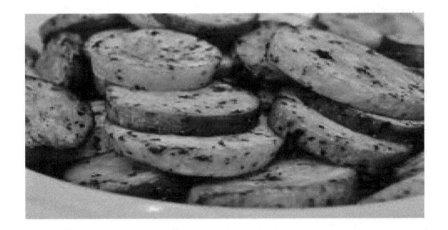

Sweets

Almond Flour Chocolate Chip Cookies
These Vegan Almond Flour Chocolate Chip Cookies are Paleo, Low-Carb, Sugar-free, easy 6-ingredient healthy cookies with only 5.8g net carbs per cookie.

Prep Time: 10 mins Cook Time: 12 mins Total Time: 22 mins

Ingredients

2 cups Almond Flour also known as almond flour or ground almond

1/4 cup Coconut oil melted

1/4 cup Sugar-free flavored maple syrup or liquid sweetener of choice (maple syrup if paleo or vegan)

1/4 teaspoon Salt + extra to sprinkle on top (optional) 1/2 teaspoon Baking soda

1/3 cup Sugar-free Chocolate Chips or >85% cocoa 2 teaspoons Vanilla extract

Instructions

Preheat oven to 180°C (350°F).

Line a cookie sheet with parchment paper. Set aside.

In a large mixing bowl add almond meal, liquid sweetener, melted coconut oil, vanilla, salt, and baking soda.

Combine with a spatula or a spoon until all the ingredients are combined and it forms pieces/crumble of cookie dough.

Use your hands to bring the pieces together into a large cookie dough ball. The dough is soft, easy to bring together into a ball, not a crumbly dough.

Roll the dough ball into a cylinder of about 20 cm long (7 inches long), use a sharp knife to divide the cylinder into 8 even pieces. I usually make 8 medium size cookies but feel free to make 6 large cookies if preferred!

Take a piece of dough, roll into a ball and place the cookie dough ball on the cookie sheet. Repeat for the other pieces of dough. Leave about a thumb space between each cookie dough ball – the cookies won't expand much when baking so you don't need lots of space between balls. Repeat for all cookie balls until you obtain 8 cookie balls on the cookie sheet covered with parchment paper.

Flatten each cookie ball with your hands. The more you press the thinner and crispier they will be. Don't press too much for a softer, chewier, and thicker cookie. If the border slightly cracks, simply use your finger to smooth the border and reshape.

Add a few dark chocolate chunks or chips onto each flattened cookies. Slightly press to stick the chocolate to the dough- not much as you don't want the chips/chunks to go through the dough. Place the chocolate chunks away from the border, to prevent the chocolate from overflowing from the cookie when baking.

Bake 12 minutes or until the edges are golden.

They will be slightly soft when out of the oven, cool down 5 minutes on the baking sheet then using a spatula, transfer onto a cooling rack.

Store for 1 week in a cookie jar.

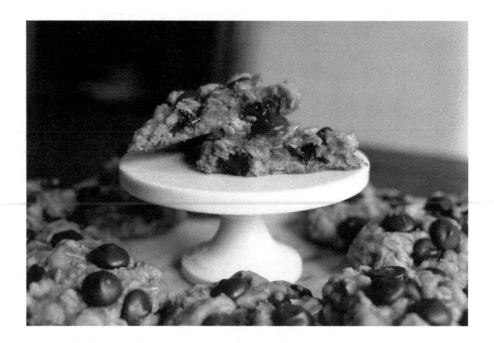

Keto Coconut cookies

Prep Time: 10 mins Cook Time: 15 mins Total Time: 25 mins

Ingredients

2 cup unsweetened desiccated coconut 200g 1 1/2 cup Almond Flour 160g

2 large Egg or 2 flax eggs if vegan 1/2 cup Coconut oil melted, or butter 1/2 cup Erythritol (100g)

1 teaspoon Vanilla essence Cookies decoration

1 teaspoons unsweetened desiccated coconut toasted if desired

Instructions

Preheat oven to 180°C (360°F). Lay a cookie sheet with baking paper. Set aside.

In a food processor, with the S blade attachment, add all the cookie ingredients.

Process on medium speed until all the ingredients come together. Scoop out the dough with a cookie scoop, and roll into a ball with your hands

Place each cookie ball on the baking tray covered with baking paper. You should be able to make 10 large cookies with the whole batter.

Press each ball with your fingers to form thick flat round cookies - about 1 cm thickness.

Bake at 180°C (360°F) for 18-23 minutes or until the sides and top are golden-brown.

Cool down on the cookie sheet for 20 minutes, they will harden slightly when cooling down.

Storage

Transfer onto a cookie rack to fully cool down to room temperature.

Store up to 5 days in a cookie jar or freeze for later.

Nutrition Info

Calories 190 Calories from Fat 107 Fat 11.9g Carbohydrates 6.3g Fiber 2.2g Sugar 1.4g Protein 4.5g

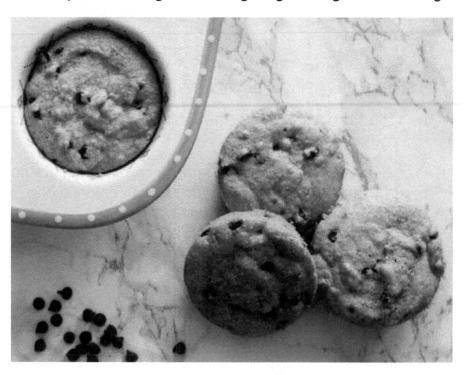

Cookie dough bars no bake, keto, vegan

Cookie Dough Bars are delicious no-bake peanut butter chocolate chips bars made with only 5 wholesome ingredients. A healthy 100% keto, low-carb, sugar-free, gluten-free, and vegan bar ready in only 30 minutes to fix a sweet craving with no guilt.

Prep Time: 10 mins Total Time: 30 mins

Ingredients

3/4 cup Almond Flour or almond flour 2 tablespoons Coconut Flour

1/2 cup Natural Peanut butter unsalted, fresh, runny 2 tablespoons Sugar-free flavored maple syrup

1/3 cup Sugar-free Chocolate Chips Chocolate nut butter layer

3 oz Sugar-free Dark Chocolate

2 tablespoons Natural Peanut butter unsalted, fresh, runny

Instructions

In a medium bowl combine the liquid sweetener and peanut butter.

Microwave 30 seconds - it will be slightly warm, stir to combine. Set aside.

Add the almond flour, coconut flour, and chocolate chips.

Stir until fully incorporated. It will form a dough that you can easily shape as a cookie dough ball.

Transfer the dough into a rectangle loaf baking pan covered with a piece of parchment paper. (my loaf pan is a 9-inch x 5- inch x 1.8-inch pan)

Press the dough with your hands to cover all the bottom of the pan. Use a spatula to make the surface flat and smooth. Freeze while you prepare the chocolate layer.

In a bowl combine the sugar-free dark chocolate and nut butter. Melt by 30 seconds bursts in the microwave stirring between to prevent the chocolate from burning. It should not require more than 90 seconds. Stir well to combine and form a shiny melted chocolate mixture.

Remove the loaf pan from the freezer, pour the melted chocolate onto the bar. Use a spatula to spread the layer evenly. Freeze again for 10-15 minutes or until the chocolate layer is set.

Cut into bars using a sharp knife. You can warm the knife blade slightly to make the cutting even easier. This recipe makes 8 square bars.

Store the bars in the fridge in an airtight plastic container or plastic bag for up to 10 days!

Nutrition Info

Calories 198 Calories from Fat 149 Fat 16.5g25% Carbohydrates 9.9g Fiber 3.9g Sugar 3g3% Protein 7.2g

Paleo Pumpkin Brownies

Prep Time: 10 mins Cook Time: 25 mins Total Time: 55 mins 16 brownie squares

Ingredients

Paleo Pumpkin Brownies

1 cup Pumpkin Puree , canned, no sugar added

1 cup almond butter , smooth, fresh, no added sugar, no added oil (or use peanut butter)

1/2 cup Sugar-free flavored maple syrup or maple syrup (if not sugar free)

1 teaspon Vanilla extract

1 teaspoon pumpkin pie spices

1 cup unsweetened cocoa powder

1/3 cup Sugar-free Chocolate Chips or dark chocolate chips 85% cocoa

Pumpkin glazing

1/3 cup almond butter , smooth, fresh, no added sugar, no added oil (or use peanut butter)

1 tablespoon Coconut oil , melted

1 tablespoon Pumpkin Puree ,canned, no sugar added 1/4 teaspoon pumpkin pie spices

1-2 Monk Fruit Drops or Stevia Drops - optional Chocolate drizzle

2 oz Sugar-free Chocolate Chips or dark chocolate 85% cocoa 1/2 teaspoon Coconut oil

Instructions

Preheat oven to 180C (350F).

Line a square brownie pan with parchment paper. Set aside.

In a food processor, using the S blade attachment add the pumpkin puree, almond butter, sugar free maple flavored syrup, pumpkin spices and vanilla.

Blend on high speed for 30 seconds or until it forms a consistent batter with a lovely orange color.

Add unsweetened cocoa powder and blend again for 30 seconds until it forms a thick, sticky and shiny brownie batter.

Stir in the chocolate chips using a spatula or the pulse mode of your food processor.

Transfer the brownie batter into the prepared brownie pan and spread evenly using a silicone spatula. The batter is sticky and that is what you want.

Sprinkle extra sugar free chocolate chips on top. Lightly press them into the batter using the spatula.

Bake for 20-25 minutes or until the top and edge are set. Remove from the oven, let cool down 15 minutes into the brownie pan.

Transfer onto a cooling rack. Meanwhile prepare the pumpkin glaze.

Pumpkin glaze

In a medium mixing bowl, add nut butter, melted coconut oil, pumpkin spices, pumpkin puree and pumpkin stevia drops.

Combine with a spoon until it forms a creamy glazing.

Drizzle on top of the cool brownie until no more left. The glazing won't harden it will stay moist and soft.

Chocolate drizzle - optional

In a microwave safe bowl, melt the sugar free chocolate chips with melted coconut oil. Microwave by 30 seconds burst, stir and repeat until fully melted. Drizzle on top of the pumpkin glazing.

You can freeze the brownie 10 minutes to set the chocolate drizzle and add an extra fudgy texture to the brownie.

Store the brownie for up to 4 days in the fridge using a cake box to prevent the brownie to dry. You can also store at room temperature up to 2 days.

Brownie can be freeze in zip bags.

Nutrition Info

Calories 154.5 Calories from Fat 120 Fat 13.3g20% Saturated Fat 2.2g Sodium 3.4mg0% Potassium 269.3mg8% Carbohydrates 8.4g3% Fiber 4.4g18% Sugar 1.6g2% Protein 5.6g

No bake peanut butter bars healthy

No bake peanut butter bars healthy dessert made with 6 simple ingredients, 100% sugar-free, gluten-free and vegan. A delicious easy low-carb recipe to fix your sweet cravings with no sugar in less than 20 minutes.

Prep Time: 15 mins Total Time: 35 mins 12 bars

Ingredients

Peanut butter layer

1 cup Natural Peanut butter unsalted, no oil added (265g) 2/3 cup Coconut Flour (72g)

1/3 cup Sugar-free powdered sweetener or powdered monk fruit/stevia blend (53g)

Chocolate Peanut butter layer

1/3 cup unsweetened cocoa powder

2 tablepoon Natural Peanut butter unsalted, no added oil or sugar (30ml)

4 tablespoon Coconut oil , melted (60ml)

2 tablespoon Sugar-free powdered sweetener

Instructions

In a medium mixing bowl, add peanut butter, coconut flour and powdered sugar-free sweetener of your choice.

Combine with a spatula, then knead with your hand to form a consistent peanut butter dough.

Transfer the peanut butter dough into a rectangle loaf baking pan covered with a piece of parchment paper. I used a cake loaf pan size: 9 inches x 5 inches X 1.8 inches.

Press the dough to cover the bottom of the pan evenly. Use a spatula to smooth the top.

Put the pan in the freezer while you prepare the chocolate peanut butter layer.

In a small mixing bowl add peanut butter and coconut oil. Microwave 30 seconds, or bring on the stove for 1 minute under low heat, stirring constantly to combine both ingredients. Stir in powdered sugar-free sweetener and unsweetened cocoa powder. Make sure you stir the mixture fast to avoid any lumps or otherwise gradually add the powdered ingredients stirring after each addition.

Remove the loaf pan from the freezer. Spread the chocolate layer on top of the peanut butter layer. It should set really fast as your base is very cold. Spread evenly using a spatula.

Freeze 30 minutes before slicing into 12 slices. Warm the knife blade under heat before cutting, it prevents the chocolate layer from breaking.

Storage

These bars are soft and must be stored in an airtight container in the fridge. Can store up to 4 weeks or freeze and eat frozen or defrost 30 minutes-1 hour before eating.

Fruity Neapolitan lolly loaf

Prep: 25 mins 25 mins plus 8 hours freezing time Easy
Serves 8

Ingredients

200g peaches nectarines or apricots (or a mixture),
stoned

200g strawberries or raspberries (or a mixture), hulled

450ml double cream

½ x 397g can condensed milk

2 tsp vanilla extract orange and pink food colouring
(optional)

8 wooden lolly sticks

Directions:

Put the peaches, nectarines or apricots in a food
processor and pulse until they're chopped and juicy but
still with some texture. Scrape into a bowl. Repeat with
the berries and scrape into another bowl.

Pour the cream, condensed milk and vanilla into a third
bowl and whip until just holding soft peaks. Add roughly
a third of the mixture to the peaches and another third
to the berries, and mix until well combined. Add a drop
of orange food colouring to the peach mixture and a drop
of pink food colouring to the berry mixture if you want a
vibrant colour. Line a 900g loaf tin or terrine mould with
cling film (look for a long thin one, ours was 23 x 7 x
8cm), then pour in the berry mixture. Freeze for 2 hrs
and chill the remaining mixtures in the fridge.

Once the bottom layer is frozen, remove the vanilla mixture from the fridge and pour over the berry layer. The bottom layer should now be firm enough to support your lolly sticks, so place these, evenly spaced, along the length of the loaf tin, pushing down gently until they stand up straight. Return to the freezer for another 2 hrs.

Once the vanilla layer is frozen, pour over the peach mixture, easing it around the lolly sticks. Return to the freezer for a further 4 hrs or until completely frozen. Remove from the freezer 10 mins before serving. Use the cling film to help you remove the loaf from the tin. Take to the table on a board and slice off individual lollies for your guests. Any leftovers can be kept in the freezer for up to 2 weeks.

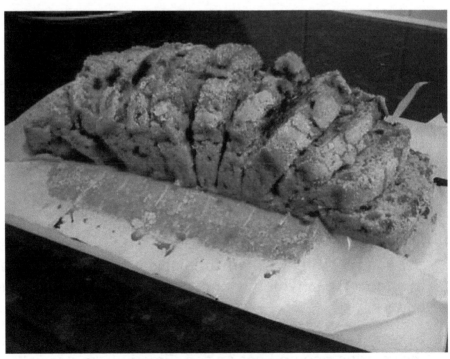

Keto Breakfast Brownie Muffins

Servingss 6

Ingredients

1 cup golden flaxseed meal ¼ cup cocoa powder 1 tablespoon cinnamon

½ tablespoon baking powder ½ teaspoon salt 1 large egg

2 tablespoons coconut oil ¼ cup sugar-free caramel syrup ½ cup pumpkin puree 1 teaspoon vanilla extract

1 teaspoon apple cider vinegar ¼ cup slivered almonds

Instructions

Preheat your oven to 350°F and combine all your dry ingredients in a deep mixing bowl and mix to combine.

In a separate bowl, combine all your wet ingredients.

Pour your wet ingredients into your dry ingredients and mix very well to combine.

Line a muffin tin with paper liners and spoon about ¼ cup of batter into each muffin liner. This recipe should Servings 6 muffins. Then sprinkle slivered almonds over the top of each muffin and press gently so that they adhere.

Bake in the oven for about 15 minutes. You should see the muffins rise and set on top. Enjoy warm or cool!

Walnut Cardamom Bar Cookies

Prep time: 20 min Cooking Time: 30 min serve: 2

Ingredients

¼ tablespoon butter, softened

½ tablespoon honey

1 egg, separated

½ tablespoon vanilla extract

1 cup coconut flour

½ teaspoon cardamom

½ teaspoon salt

½ tablespoon chopped walnut

½ tablespoons Butter

¼ teaspoon vanilla extract

1 tablespoon coconut milk, or as needed

Instructions

Grease a pan.

In a large bowl, cream together 1cup of butter, honey and light and fluffy. Mix in the egg yolk and vanilla. Combine the coconut flour, cardamom and salt; stir into the batter until it forms a soft dough. Spread evenly in the prepared pan. Brush the top with egg white and sprinkle walnut over the top.

Pour the water into the Instant Pot Insert, and place a trivet with the covered brownie cake tin into the Instant Pot.

Cover your Instant Pot, set the vent to Sealing, select the Manual or pressure cook button, select high pressure and set the timer to 20 mins.

When done allow the pot to undergo natural pressure release for 15 mins

Nutrition Facts

Calories 155, Total Fat 7.7g, Saturated Fat 3.5g, Cholesterol 93mg, Sodium 644mg, Total Carbohydrate

20.5g, Dietary Fiber 0.3g , Total Sugars 19.7g, Protein 3.4g

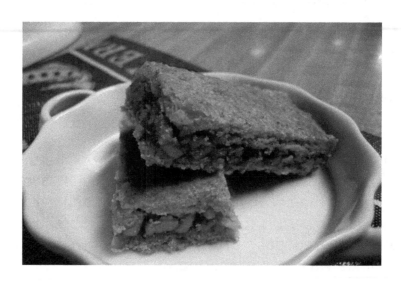

Lemon-Lime Magic Cake

Prep time: 20 min Cooking Time: 40 min serve: 2

Ingredients Cake Layer

½ cup almond flour

1 cup coconut milk

½ cup butter melted

2 eggs

Lemon-Lime Layer

2 eggs, slightly beaten

1 tablespoon honey

1 tablespoon finely grated lemon peel

1 tablespoon finely grated lime peel

¼ tablespoon fresh lemon juice

¼ tablespoon fresh lime juice

Topping

1 container (4 Oz) Cool Whip frozen whipped topping, thawed

Instructions

Cake Layer:

In large bowl, beat almond flour, coconut milk, butter and eggs with electric mixer on medium speed 2 minutes, scraping bowl occasionally. Pour in pan. 3. Lemon-Lime

Layer: In another large bowl, mix eggs, honey, lemon peel, lemon juice, lime peel and lime juice.

Pour the water into the Instant Pot Insert, and place a trivet with the covered brownie cake tin into the Instant Pot.

Cover your Instant Pot, set the vent to Sealing, select the manual or pressure cook button, select high pressure and set the timer to 30 minutes.

When done allow the pot to undergo natural pressure release for 15 mins

Cool 30 mins. Refrigerate at least 4 hours to chill. Spread whipped topping over chilled cake. Sprinkle with additional lemon and lime peel if desired. Using a serving spatula and a knife to help slide pieces off carefully,

Serve and enjoy

Nutrition Facts

Calories 453, Total Fat 37.4g, Saturated Fat 28.1g, Cholesterol 327mg , Sodium 142mg, Total Carbohydrate 16.6g, Dietary Fiber 2.9g , Total Sugars 13.5g, Protein 14g

Vanilla Pudding

Prep time: 25 min Cooking Time: 15 min serve: 2

Ingredients

1 tablespoon maple syrup 1 tablespoon corn starch 1/8 teaspoon salt

2 cups coconut milk 1 large egg yolks

½ tablespoon unsalted butter 1 teaspoon pure vanilla extract

Instructions

In an Instant Pot, combine maple syrup, corn-starch, salt, coconut milk, and egg yolks. Cover your Instant Pot, set the vent to Sealing, select the manual or pressure cook button, select high pressure and set the timer to 5 minutes.

When done allow the pot to undergo natural pressure release for 15 mins

About 8-10 minutes. Note: It will thicken more as it cools.

Place a fine mesh strainer over a large heatproof bowl. Pour the mixture through the strainer and into the bowl.

Transfer the pudding from the large bowl or into individual serving bowls.

Cool slightly, then cover with plastic wrap. Refrigerate for several hours or until chilled.

Little Jam Tarts

Prep:15 mins Cook:15 mins Easy Makes 20

Ingredients

500g sweet shortcrust pastry

20 tsp jam (we used apricot, blackcurrant and strawberry)

Directions:

Roll out the shortcrust pastry on a lightly floured surface to just under the thickness of £1 coin. Stamp out 20 x 5cm circles using a pastry cutter and line 2 mini muffin tins (or make in 2 batches).

Prick with a fork and spoon 1 tsp jam into each (we used apricot, blackcurrant and strawberry). Stamp out shapes from the leftover pastry to decorate the tarts, if you like.

Bake at 200C/180C fan/gas 6 for 12-15 mins, until the pastry is golden.

Macadamia & Cranberry American Cookies

Prep: 20 mins Cook:12 mins easy Makes 55

Ingredients

3 x 200g/7oz white chocolate bars, chopped

200g butter

2 eggs

100g light muscovado sugar

175g golden caster sugar

2 tsp vanilla extract

350g plain flour

2 tsp baking powder

1 tsp cinnamon

100g dried cranberry

100g macadamia nut, chopped

Directions:

Heat oven to 180C/160C fan/gas 4. Melt 170g of the chocolate, then allow to cool. Beat in the butter, eggs, sugars and vanilla, preferably with an electric hand whisk, until creamy. Stir in the flour, baking powder, cinnamon and cranberries with two-thirds of the remaining chocolate and macadamias, to make a stiff dough.

Using a tablespoon measure or a small ice-cream scoop, drop small mounds onto a large baking dish, spacing them well apart, then poke in the reserved chocolate, nuts and berries. Bake in batches for 12 mins until pale golden, leave to harden for 1-2 mins, then cool on a wire rack.

Freeze, open-freeze the raw cookie dough scoops on baking trays; when solid, pack them into a freezer container, interleaving the layers with baking parchment. Use within 3 months. Bake from frozen for 15-20 mins.

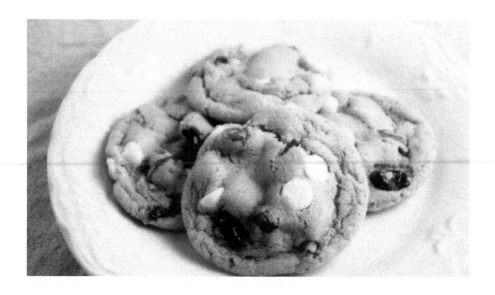

Lightning Source UK Ltd.
Milton Keynes UK
UKHW021359070521
383304UK00001B/67